PEARL FAGAN

The Wonders of Chiropractic

Unbreak Your Back and Revitalize Your Spirit

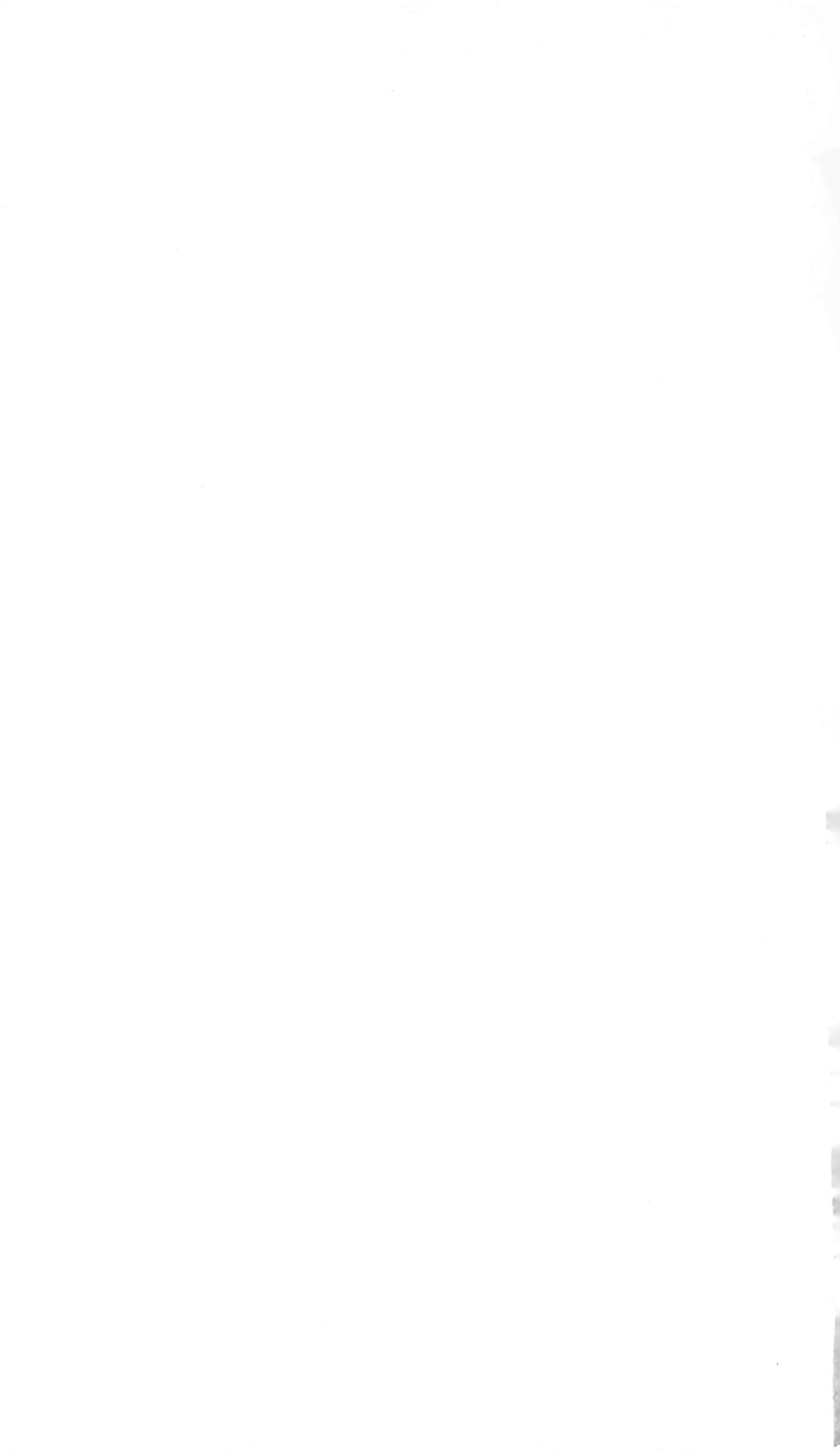

First edition

Contents

1

Introduction

In the fast-paced rhythm of our modern lives, where stress and sedentary habits often take a toll on our bodies, there exists an ancient art that has stood the test of time — Chiropractic. Welcome to a journey of discovery, a guide to unlocking the profound benefits that lie within the realm of chiropractic care.

In "The Wonders of Chiropractic," we embark on a quest to unburden our backs and reignite the spirit that resides within. This book is more than a compilation of facts; it celebrates the remarkable ways chiropractic practices can transform lives. As we delve into the pages ahead, we'll unravel the mysteries surrounding Chiropractic, exploring its various types, techniques, and the science behind its profound impact on well-being.

Join me in uncovering the wisdom passed down through generations, the hands that heal, and the science that harmonizes body and spirit. Whether you're a skeptic seeking answers or a seasoned chiropractic patient, this journey promises revelations that will resonate with your body, mind, and soul.

But who the heck am I to say?

Well, let me start by saying, 'Chiropractic Saved My Life.' It really did; my only wish is that I had known then what I know now. Before you can understand how it saved my life, you first must know why it needed saving!

In my 17th year of life, I took some hard hits physically. I loved, and still do love, doing 'extreme' sports, but when I was 17, those sports did not love me back. In fact, they nearly put me in a wheelchair. In the summer of my 17th year, in the 1990s, I fell off my horse when I incorrectly anticipated his moves after being startled. I expected the first movement sideways but did not expect the leapfrog forward after that. Which left me up in the air about 5.5 feet from the hard-grade gravel road that I slammed onto, flat on my lower back.

As you can guess, I did what I was always told to do - 'Get back up on that horse' and tough it out. I was able to tough it out and ride my horse home the final 2 miles it took, but by the time I got there, I couldn't move, and the pain was astronomical. I had to fall off the saddle into my parents' arms to be carried into the house.

The doctor's visits began. Starting with our general practitioner and then moving on to an orthopedic doctor, spinal specialist/-surgeon, and physical therapist. The fall had caused two of my lower vertebrae to twist, forcing the spinous process sideways. To make things even more complicated, one vertebrae twisted to the left and the other to the right.

Ultimately, they said I needed surgery - pins in my back to hold the vertebrae in place so they wouldn't twist anymore. Due to my age and the current medical advancements of the 1990s, we opted OUT of having me go under the knife. They told us that if I didn't get pins in my back or go through with the surgery, I would be in a wheelchair by the time I was 30. At the time, we felt that back surgery was a guaranteed life of pain, but the injury might have a chance of improvement, even though we didn't know how.

So, as an alternative, I went through lots of physical therapy to help me regain some of my mobility, along with the use of electro-stim therapy for the surrounding muscles and the very well-known pain management treatment (i.e., heavy prescription pain blockers).

In that same year of my youth, flash forward to winter; I was on the slopes, shredding powder! I loved skiing! My dad taught me from a very young age, so I loved the challenge of going through trees, off jumps, and as fast as possible! I had no fear. Although my back hurt, I was happy on the slopes and could push that pain to the back of my mind and enjoy the rush.

One particular day, I was racing a friend down the designated racing slope, but it had yet to be combed. That meant it wasn't packed down to cover the ground, and it was all powder to be fluffed by the turning of my skis! Until one of those turns had my skis hitting a rock (which would typically be covered if the slope had been combed), I had the grandest of yard sales. My stuff went everywhere. I knew when I hit that rock that this was going to be a bad one, and then I lost consciousness. Upon waking, I had my friend by my side as well as my brother-in-law, who had run back UP the slope to get to me.

I remember them both being highly attentive and oddly calm, telling me ski patrol was on the way and **not to move**. It was apparent to them that something in the fall had caused the circulation on the left side of my body to cease, not permanently, but enough that the left side of my face had lost all color and instantly withered. When ski patrol arrived, they put me in a neck brace and brought me down the slope in an emergency sled, where we were met by an ambulance.

The ER took x-rays and determined that it was just a hairline fracture and would heal independently, as long as I was careful. And although the fracture may have 'healed,' there was still a lot of pain. My neck was never quite the same after that, nor was my overall health. The combination of injuries I sustained were livable without surgical intervention, though riddled with pain. But pain can be masked, and symptoms can be addressed as they arise. That is precisely what I did, but what I didn't know was that these injuries, the pain 'management' methods, and treating the symptoms were doing way more damage to my body and mind than I ever realized.

For the 6 years following that most unfortunate year of my youth, I dealt with mysterious illnesses, unusual ailments, and, of course, all that pain. I was in and out of hospitals, doctors' offices, physical therapists, and pain management doctors. I had x-rays, MRIs, CT scans, blood tests, biopsies, EKG, spinal tap, EEG, you name it. So many tests, guesses, and 'pseudo-diagnosis', but yet, I had very few answers.

At 23 years old, I was taking several different types of medication. My back & neck pain were given, but then they couldn't explain why my head hurt all the time. They'd say cluster headaches, allergy headaches, stress headaches, because of hormones, because of depression, it just kept going, and I never got any resolution other than more drugs to mask it all. The issue with all of that was that I was also masking who I was; it altered my brain, and I did NOT like it. The headaches were preferred over the zombie effect I was getting.

So, I tried the one alternative medical option I wasn't completely terrified of - massage therapy. Oh, it felt so good for that one hour I was on the table. Sadly, it didn't last, and I started going more frequently. Finally, one day, my masseuse told me he could only do so much because it wasn't the muscles that were the root problem; instead, it was my neck and overall spinal structure. I needed to see a chiropractor. Those words hit me like a freaky freight train. I'd seen a friend get adjusted by a quackipractor once, and it was traumatizing. Regardless, I let the term 'root problem' rattle around in my brain as I contemplated the world of Chiropractic.

When I returned to work that day as a receptionist, I got a call from a telemarketer informing me of a special at a local Chiropractic office. All I needed to do was bring in some canned food for people experiencing homelessness, and I would get my first exam, x-rays, and treatment at no cost. That was my sign. So, I signed up and went in.

That is how Chiropractic saved my life as I finally embarked on my healing journey!

There is much about this journey that I want to share with you. However, that might take more than one book! Thus, the following chapters will walk you through the basics of what I've learned over the last 20 years, all lumped together in a concise and tear-free manner. Trust me, I've already cried all the tears, and now you can benefit from the reservoir of my results and learn how Chiropractic unbroke my back and revitalized my spirit!

Are you ready to break free from the constraints of discomfort and embrace the revitalizing wonders of Chiropractic? Let the exploration begin.

2

Today's Spinal Healthcare

The Spine

The spine is the very core of the skeletal structure, providing general shape, body posture, flexibility, and movement to twist and bend. A healthy spine will have 3 natural s-shaped curves that act as shock absorbers. In conjunction with the curves, facet joints and disks rest between each vertebra, assisting with shock absorption and the ability to move and twist at each vertebral joint.

Soft tissues such as ligaments, tendons, and muscles surround the spine to aid with movement and help prevent injury. Then there is the spinal cord, containing 32 pairs of nerve clusters that branch out through the vertebrae into the rest of the body.

The spine is made up of 5 distinct segments. The spine starts from the top, where the skull rests on the Atlas bone.

1 - The 1st segment is **the Cervical spine** (vertebrae C1 to vertebrae C7), the neck region. The cervical spine makes an inward C-shape called a lordotic curve, allowing one to turn, tilt, and nod their head.

2 - The 2nd segment is **the Thoracic spine** (vertebrae T1 to vertebrae T12), the middle back region, and the largest segment, and is where the ribs stem from. This segment bends out slightly, making a backward C-shape called a kyphotic curve.

3 - The 3rd segment is **the Lumbar spine** (vertebrae L1 to vertebrae L5), and it supports the upper structure of the spine. The Lumbar region also connects the pelvis and bears most of the body weight and the stress of lifting and carrying items. The Lumbar region is the most commonly injured segment of the spine. The lumbar segment bends inward, creating a C-shaped lordotic curve.

4 - The 4th segment is **the Sacrum** (vertebrae S1 to vertebrae S5), which is 5 vertebrae fused together during fetal development. This fused spine segment connects to the hips, creating the 'pelvic girdle.'

5 - The 5th and final segment is **the Coccyx**, also known as the tailbone, which is 4 fused vertebrae at the bottom of the spine.

Now that we know the basics of the spinal structure, we will look at the importance of the cargo (aka the nerves) that the spinal cord carries within it.

The Neurology

Nerves send electrical impulses back and forth between the brain and other body parts to help feel sensations and engage muscle movement. Nerves also control autonomic body functions such as digestion, maintaining heart rate, breathing & regulation, and so on. All of these nerves and nerve impulses travel through the spine. The rate of travel is truly astronomical. If you stub your toe, that sensation is transmitted from your toe into your brain within milliseconds, and your cry out in pain appears to be simultaneous with the action. That's fast!

But what if there is a breakdown in that communication? Say you stub your toe but don't get any warning from your brain that it hurts. You will keep moving about your day; all the while, your toe is getting increasingly larger due to inflammation that you would have taken care of had your nervous system adequately notified you. How on earth could something like that happen?

Well, imagine the spine as a 33-mile underwater superhighway with hundreds of lanes of traffic going in two different directions. Along the first 26 miles are 32 exits and entrances, and no HOV or carpool lane exists. Usually, this is a very well-oiled machine, and traffic flows freely and swiftly. Every vehicle (nerve) has a defined destination. Every driver (nerve impulse) knows where it needs to go and how to get there. But when there is a disruption in the flow of traffic, the entire underwater superhighway is affected, and everything slows down and goes into fight or flight mode. That would be similar to a minor spinal issue such as a pulled muscle, strain in the neck or back, etc.

However, if there is a traffic accident, most traffic will come to a temporary halt, the exits and entrances will get jammed up, and most of those on the highway will not reach their destination on time. Some may even end up at the wrong destination in an attempt to circumvent the accident, which can only be done by taking the wrong exit. Signals get crossed, information gets missed or lost, more accidents could occur, and so much more. Once the accident has been addressed and things are cleared off the highway, getting the highway travelers back to that original speed limit will still take time. Some may have gotten cut off, others are misguided, and those in the accident need immediate care.

In the hustle and bustle of it all, we only worry about fixing the symptoms that require immediate attention. Then, we just stop until the next traffic accident or signal from the superhighway deems more work is needed. Even then, these signals could point at just another symptom we wouldn't typically associate with a spinal issue being the root cause.

Next is a graph of the spine that breaks down the different segments, the individual vertebrae, and what part of your body each nerve cluster is communicating with as it leaves the spine through the facet joints.

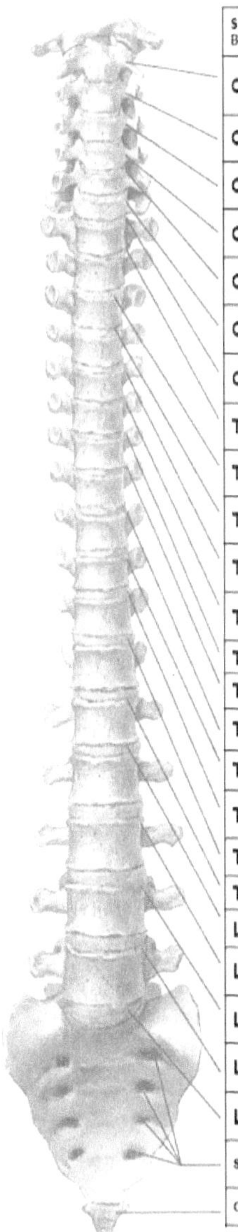

Spinal Bone	Nerve Supply	Common Warning Signs
C1	Blood supply to the head, pituitary gland, scalp, bones of the face, brain, inner ear and middle ear.	• Headaches •insomnia •high blood pressure • Migraines • chronic fatigue • dizziness
C2	Eyes, ears, sinuses, tongue, forehead	• Sinusitis • ear aches • pain around the eyes • Vision problems • hearing problems
C3	Cheeks, outer ear, face bones, teeth, facial nerves	• Neuralgia • pimples • eczema
C4	Nose, lips, mouth, Eustachian tube	• Hay fever • runny nose • hearing loss • Adenoids
C5	Vocal cords, neck, glands, pharynx	• Sore throat • laryngitis • hoarseness
C6	Neck muscles, shoulders, tonsils	• Stiff neck • arm pain • tonsillitis • Persistent cough
C7	Thyroid gland, shoulder bursa, elbows	• Bursitis • colds • thyroid conditions
T1	Forearms, hands, wrists, fingers, esophagus, trachea	• Arm and hand pain • difficulty breathing • shortness of breath • asthma
T2	Heart, coronary arteries	• Heart conditions • chest conditions
T3	Lungs, bronchial tubes, pleura, chest	• Bronchitis • pleurisy • pneumonia • congestion
T4	Gallbladder	• Gallbladder conditions • jaundice • shingles
T5	Liver, solar plexus, circulation	• Liver conditions • blood pressure conditions • poor circulation
T6	Stomach	• Indigestion • heartburn • dyspepsia
T7	Pancreas, duodenum	• Ulcers • gastritis
T8	Spleen	• Lower resistance
T9	Adrenal glands	• Allergies • chronic fatigue
T10	Kidneys	• Kidney problems • hardening of the arteries • fatigue • nephritis
T11	Kidneys, ureters	• Skin conditions • eczema • pimples
T12	Small intestines, lymph circulation	• Rheumatism • gas pains
L1	Large intestines, inguinal rings	• Colitis • diarrhea • hernia
L2	Appendix, abdomen, thigh	• Cramps • varicose veins • leg pain
L3	Sex organs, uterus, bladder, knees	• Menstrual pains • irregular periods • miscarriages • impotency • knee pain
L4	Prostate gland, lower back	• Back pain • difficulty, painful or frequent urination
L5	Lower back, buttocks, thighs, legs, feet, sciatic nerve, large intestine	• Back pain • leg pain •constipation
Sacrum	Hip bones, buttocks	• Sacroiliac conditions • back pain • hip pain
Coccyx	Rectum, anus	• Hemorrhoids • tail bone pain

The Pain and The Relief

Not everyone, thankfully, has had a major accident that damaged their spine, such as I have. But a twinge here, a tweak there, a pinch on that side, a shooting pain down the hip, a pull across the shoulders, tightness at the bra line, sore neck; at some point, everybody experiences spinal pain.

There are varying degrees of back pain and personal tolerances. A majority of people who experience mild back pain can ignore it or take over-the-counter medication until it subsides. They could be doing that once a year, once a month, or more frequently. But it is a mild pain, so it isn't bad enough for one to raise any concern about it with a doctor.

Then you have the folks that have persistent, nagging pain. This degree of pain is usually a constant thing that is easily masked by over-the-counter medications and temporarily eased with stretching and exercise.

Last is the back pain attributed to things such as scoliosis, congenital malformation, or a direct injury. People suffering from pain of this degree typically know why they are hurting and usually seek professional care. Whether that is a family practitioner, another medical specialist, physical or massage therapist, or so on, they are actively seeking or maintaining a level of treatment.

The Domino Effect

The one thing that all these degrees of pain have in common is that they ALL directly affect the nervous system. Remember that underwater superhighway with all those exits and entrances? Imagine if one of the sections (vertebra) between two exits gets shifted or twisted somehow. The exits on either side of this portion of the superhighway will now be askew. Although travelers can still get through, it is a bumpy ride that can rattle the driver, much like a twisted vertebra can cause the nerve impulses to falter.

Most people don't realize – back pain or not – that everything in the body is directly or indirectly affected by the overall functionality of the superhighway (spine). So, if your back hurts, just think about other symptoms you might have that could be associated with a misalignment in your spine. Maybe one has cold feet, tingly fingers, Irritable Bowel Syndrome, frequent headaches, acid reflux, etc., which could be the direct result of spinal misalignment and, in turn, could be helped or corrected with the right kind of intervention.

If you recall, I mentioned how my injuries were causing more than I ever realized. Well, this is what I mean by the domino effect. I was injured in my 17th year, and I chose not to do surgery; rather, I went with physical therapy and medication. Oof. In my 18th year, I had what appeared to be a stroke. The entire left side of my body was on fire, yet unmovable. I was in heaps of pain from my eyeballs down to my toes. I was in the E.R. for several hours, getting poked, prodded, and questioned.

That day, I learned about the joys of spinal taps, EEGs, and EKGs. By the end of the visit, I was told that <u>nothing was wrong with me</u> according to their tests, and there were a lot of tests.

It was a painful recovery from the spinal tap as my body had to replenish the fluid that ran through my brain and spinal cord. Per the E.R. instructions, if I still felt ill after that 2-week recovery, I should go back to my primary care doctor. I did that and was promptly put on an IV and then pumped full of antibiotics and anti-inflammatories after their tests finally revealed Sinusitis, Bronchitis, Tendonitis in both my left shoulder and my left hip, and Inflamed Bowel Disorder. To put it simply, I *was* on fire! I had massive inflammation throughout the entire left side of my body, and my nervous system and immune system were overloaded.

Although I got the treatment I needed for all of these ailments, they couldn't explain WHY that all happened at once and why on such a grand scale. I spent a month of my senior year of high school on bedrest without any real answers. Back then, 'root cause' wasn't something we considered - it was about fixing the symptom(s) at hand. And boy, those symptoms kept rolling in. At the time, I had no idea that all of these issues were offshoots of the root problem: my improperly-treated neck and back injuries.

I now know that nearly all of the issues I experienced with my health from that fateful year 17 until I found chiropractic were direct effects of my injuries. Things were twisted and fractured, which caused issues with my underwater superhighway. Some exits and entrances had been blocked, pinched, twisted, and torn; the drivers could not relay their messages for autonomic body functions, and things were falling apart right under my nose.

As things fell apart, I continued to take more and more prescribed medications to treat the symptoms as they came. Anyone who has been on multiple prescriptions at a time knows that there can also be a domino effect with drug interactions, thus causing these symptomatic treatments to ultimately fail in the long run.

So, what *can* we do when it comes to spinal pain?

3

The Non-Chiropractic Alternatives

Buckle Up Buttercup: Learn to just live with the pain

Like I said earlier, you will have some folks, maybe you, that will just deal with the pain. Maybe it is so minor that they don't even notice it enough to let it bother them. Or maybe it is a bad pain, but you're the Hulk, so it doesn't matter! Usually, some OTC pain medication does the trick.

Regardless of the true pain level, the amount of over-the-counter (OTC) medications taken, or a high pain tolerance - this is not the best option. Why? The sensation of pain is your body's last resort for getting your attention to know that something is wrong. OTC medications may help with inflammation, but they will not fix the root of the pain; they only cover it up. Even just minor neck or back pain should be addressed with a chiropractor to ensure that everything is functioning properly and that there isn't a misalignment.

The Physical 'Terrorist': Learn how to move and live with less pain

First off, I want to apologize to anyone reading this who is a physical therapist - you are important, I appreciate the work that you do, and we need you! However, during my time in physical therapy, I had a Physical Terrorist who was bent on getting me unbent. They put electro-stim nodes on my muscles and used forced stretches to regain flexibility. It was a painful and non-rewarding experience as they forced my back to move in ways it hadn't ever moved, even before the accident.

Don't get me wrong, there is a time and place for physical therapy, but when it comes to your spine, a *good* chiropractor will always know best!

Under the Knife: Remove one pain but gain another

When it's necessary, surgery can be amazing, but when it isn't necessary yet still done, it usually becomes a trade-off of pains. Same place, different pain. Anytime a spinal surgery involves pins or fusion, mobility is decreased, and hopefully, some of the pain is too. However, with mobility decreased, this may be another domino effect of issues that crop up due to the immobility of separate vertebrae. That type of procedure would also greatly limit what a chiropractor can do in the future.

The main thing I would suggest here is if you get a diagnosis that requires surgery on your spine - get a second opinion and make it a trusted chiropractor!

Drugs Drugs Drugs: Masking the pain and losing your brain

There are so many medications out there that are both OTC and Prescribed that can help with inflammation and pain. As well as a slew of other drugs that get prescribed to treat the symptoms that arise from back pain. Those that help relieve the pain are simply deadening your nerve clusters and allowing the communication to flow to the brain that everything is OK. But it's NOT ok; it is a trick on your conscience brain, and the moment it fades, you're pining for the next fix. Which, again, is NOT a fix to the root of the problem!

Pain will continue to persist regardless of what you keep trying to tell your brain through medications. The root of the problem still exists and continues to degrade and miscommunicate throughout your superhighway.

I was on this horrible cycle of pain medications, and mine were way above anything you could get OTC. I had built up a tolerance to one kind, so I had to switch to another. When I built up the tolerance for that, I then had to go to something stronger, and then I was using two at a time, and it just kept coming, and my health continued to decline. At one point, I was dealing with kidney and liver stones. Did the doctors ever say that maybe it was because of all the drugs they had me on? No! They just gave me more drugs.

The Strange Way: Mindfulness and Conscience Awareness

Wouldn't it be nice if we all had the mental insight and awareness of Dr. Stephen Strange? You know, that hero-guy who healed his hands with the power of his mind and all the magic of the universe! Well, we can! Ok, maybe not all of the magic in the universe, but we can tap into the power of our minds. I don't mean to heal directly but indirectly and wholly throughout the mind and body.

Mediation and mindfulness have been long thought of as healing practices. Although it will not fix broken bones, it can help with the energy surrounding those bones. I suggest finding a body-scan meditation practice that walks you through the body-scanning process. This process is a visual practice of viewing your body as a whole, taking note of each limb and extremity, moving into the organs, soft tissues, and bones, and envisioning positive light and healthy energy surrounding every cell of your body. By doing this type of meditation regularly, one will start to notice increased blood flow, less pain, and a greater awareness of yourself.

I have come to find that using the Stephen Strange Way in conjunction with Chiropractic care has been the most beneficial to me throughout the years. Along with meditation, I also use affirmations - whether I write them down to look at them every day OR when I have to change my password, I make it a phrase that acts as an affirmation or goal. That way, I am typing it out multiple times daily, and it is always on my mind.

Some examples of affirmations for good spinal health are:

- "I nurture my spine with care and gratitude."
- "Every day, my spine grows stronger and more flexible."
- "I am aligned, balanced, and full of vitality."
- "I am grateful for the support and strength of my spine."
- "I choose movements that promote a healthy and happy spine."
- "My spine is a pillar of strength, supporting my well-being."
- "I breathe in strength, exhale tension, and support my spine."
- "I am mindful of my posture, keeping my spine aligned."
- "With each step, my spine is aligned and perfectly balanced."
- "I am kind to my spine, and it responds with strength and resilience."

Pick one, rotate through all, or develop an affirmation that resonates with you. Repeat these affirmations regularly to combine them with healthy habits such as chiropractic care for optimal spinal well-being.

4

The Chiropractic Way

What IS chiropractic?

As defined by WebMD, "Chiropractic is a healthcare profession that cares for your neuromusculoskeletal system — the bones, nerves, muscles, tendons, and ligaments. A chiropractor helps manage back and neck pain through spinal adjustments and other modalities to maintain good alignment. Chiropractic is focused on the body's ability to self-heal and includes other treatments like nutrition and exercise.'

I couldn't agree more with that definition. From my own experience of watching a friend's quackipractor 'crack her' to all the medical doctors' warnings, I honestly thought that Chiropractic was scary, dangerous, fly-by-the-night practices run by uneducated quacks and that was not at all what I was looking for.

When I got that call from the telemarketer and signed up for an appointment, I was terrified. I didn't know what to expect or what to ask. I knew nothing about the different types of chiropractors or the various adjustment modalities they use. I didn't know what level of education or certification a Chiropractor would need or if they were held accountable by a board of ethics. The 'I don't knows' kept coming. Even after I started treatment, I kept learning and healing. The best part is that I am still learning and growing every day!

Quacks versus Cracks

Just as there are many medical doctors out there with a specialty, Chiropractors will usually find their niche, too. Whether that niche is for athletics, car accidents, general practice, cervical spine only, lumbar spine only, pediatrics, prenatal, etc., they ultimately fall into one of two *types* of Chiropractor: Corrective or Relief.

Corrective

The corrective chiropractor aims to correct spinal misalignments so that the rest of your body can heal and function optimally. Corrective chiropractors typically take x-rays or spinal imaging, much like an ultrasound. They will also sit down with you to go over your concerns, review your medical history, and formulate a treatment plan that is specific to you. These types of chiropractors will not adjust your spine until they have a clear picture of your spine and your health/medical history. Each visit will be personalized; in most cases, they will assign exercises or other home remedies to utilize between visits.

Depending on the severity of your issue, you could be on an immediate treatment plan that requires several visits within a short period of time. From there, the visits would get fewer and farther apart. Or you may be in a place where just a monthly maintenance adjustment is needed.

Relief

The relief chiropractor aims to provide relief from a twinge here, a pull there, or just that sweet sweet pop. Relief chiropractors rarely do x-rays or spinal scans. They typically have an open-air office with several adjustment tables side by side. They will generally have you fill out a basic form where you mark all of your aches and pains on a skeleton. They will take a look over that, maybe ask you a couple of questions, and then have you lay face down and wait your turn to get adjusted.

Relief chiropractors are great for those folks who do not have any major issues with their spine. If it *really* is just a 'good pop' that you need, and you can inform the relief chiropractor what and how you need to be adjusted, you should be fine!

If you have trepidation about going to a chiropractor or have sustained a recent injury to your spine, this is not the chiropractor you are looking for. Going back to that superhighway concept.

If there is a breakdown in the structure, we will want a crew that does extensive research on the superhighway and they have a well-formulated plan for getting things fixed. We will not hire the crew that flew in yesterday. They have yet to see (nor do they want to see) what the issue is and just want to try fixing it.

Qualifications & Accountability

According to the National Center for Complementary and Integrative Health, chiropractors have educational and licensing standards at both national and state levels.

Those requirements are:

✓ They must earn a Doctor of Chiropractic (D.C.) degree, which the program typically takes 4 years to complete.

✓ Before enrolling in the D.C. degree program, students must have had at least 3 years of undergraduate education.

✓ The Council on Chiropractic Education accredits institutions that award the D.C. degree and is recognized as an accrediting agency by the U.S. Secretary of Education. In 2017, there were 15 accredited D.C. programs on 18 campuses.

✓ They must then pass the National Board of Chiropractic Examiners exam.

ᐁ Finally, they must obtain a state license. Many states also require chiropractors to pass an exam about state-specific laws.

<u>All states require practicing chiropractors to take continuing education classes.</u>

Chiropractic education includes classes in basic sciences, such as anatomy and physiology, and supervised clinical experience in which students learn skills such as spinal assessment, adjustment techniques, and making diagnoses. Some chiropractors complete postgraduate education in specialized fields, such as orthopedics or pediatrics.

So, believe it or not, Relief and Corrective have the same requirements to run a chiropractic practice. So why the big difference? Well, it just comes down to the chiropractor and why they got into it in the first place. In my experience, those who choose to be corrective chiropractors have generally taken additional schooling to define their niche.

One chiropractor I visited had additional education on the brain, atlas, and axis. He could perform other adjustments, but he specialized in cranial and cervical spine care, and his main objective was to relieve patients 'headaches. And not just the current headache knocking but the root of the problem causing the headaches. There is that word again: ROOT!

It is all about getting to the root cause of where all of the pain and illness is stemming from. It is not about ignoring or covering up the side effects and symptoms. The more covering up there is, the harder it is to see and address the true root cause. The vicious cycle ensues or you BREAK FREE!

Adjustment Modalities Used

Now that you know what chiropractic is and what requirements are needed for someone to practice chiropractic, what does that actually mean? What is it that chiropractors really do? Here is a list, with basic definitions, of the most popular adjustment types a chiropractor may use to correct spinal pain and injury.

The Diversified Technique has 3 main purposes. Restore spinal alignment, repair joint dysfunction, and ensure proper movement and mobility. Chiropractors use hands-on thrusts with extreme precision, restoring spinal alignment and increasing a patient's range of motion that may be affected by misaligned joints or bones. This technique is widely used, with 96% of all chiropractors using the Diversified Technique on approximately 70% of their patients.

Spinal Mobilization (aka Spinal Manipulation), also called manual therapy or spinal manipulation, is utilized by chiropractors and physical therapists alike to relieve joint pressure, reduce inflamma-tion, and improve nerve function. This technique is similar to the diversified technique discussed above but utilizes gentler thrusting motions and more stretching.

The Thompson Drop-Table technique utilizes a special table con-structed of padded platforms fitted with drop mechanisms so the patient can be "dropped" a fraction of an inch as the chiropractor applies a quick thrust to complete the adjustment. The gentle dropping motion, resembling a light vibration, is amorecomfortable option for patients. (This is one of my preferred adjustments!)

The Gonstead Adjustment *is used to restore normal disc alignment and maximum mobility. It can be administered with the patient sitting up or lying on their side. The specificity of the contact point on the chiropractor's hand plays a major role in this type of adjustment.*

The Activator *method is done via a small handheld device known as an 'Activator' to administer a gentle impulse to the extremities or the vertebral segments of the spine. The spring-loaded device is used to adjust the nervous system's tone and can treat various conditions, from headaches to lower back pain issues. (This is another one of my preferred methods.)*

The Flexion Distraction *technique utilizes a table that distracts and flexes the spine in a gentle, rhythmic movement. This technique commonly treats symptomatic disc injuries with back and leg pain. The adjustment is pain-free and even considered comfortable, making it a great option for patients with recent injuries or extra sensitivity to other types of adjustments.*

Spinal decompression *could be considered more of a chiropractic technique than an adjustment. Still, it is worth mentioning since it effectively treats lower back pain symptoms resulting from bulging, herniated, degenerated, and slipped discs. Spinal decompression utilizes a special table that carefully stretches the spine, promoting the healthy flow of water, oxygen, and other essential fluids into the discs and throughout the spine. (This is a technique that I find very fascinating, but I am not able to take advantage of this type of* *chiropractic, but that is a story for another day!*

The McKenzie Method® *is one other method that all chiropractors know about but it was actually discovered and documented by a Physiotherapist back in the 1950's. This a technique that is unique in its own right and can be utilized by a broad range of medical and alternative medicine practitioners. There are institutes around the world that are dedicated to teaching and using this method of spinal and extremity repair.*

Although it is not an official chiropractic method, I have found it beneficial in my recovery and is a daily routine for maintaining flexibility in my lower back. You can learn more about the McKenzie Method® of Mechanical Diagnosis and Therapy® institutes by searching it online or reviewing the resources at the end of this book.

As I said, that was a short list of the most popular or commonly used chiropractic techniques, but there are several that I didn't mention and have listed below for your quick reference of how many options are truly out there!

- Muscle stimulation
- Myofascial release
- Extremity manipulation
- Thompson
- Soft tissue Therapy
- Articulatory
- Functional technique
- Sacro Occipital Technique
- Ultrasound
- Chiropractic BioPhysics
- Cranial
- Ice & Heat Therapy
- Logan Basic Technique
- Release Work
- Therapeutic exercise

How to find the right chiropractor for you

Use these next couple of pages as your guide and data gatherer to finding the right chiropractor for you. **These are suggested questions to ask.** Once you have the answers, you will want to review the things that matter most to you regarding what you need from chiropractic care. Each questionnaire, follow this one, provides more insight as you get further into your journey, so do not stop here!!

One of Three Questionnaires

Name:

Number:

Address:

Days & Hours of Operation:

Is this practice Corrective or Relief Chiropractic?

Does this practice take x-rays and/or spinal scans?

Does this practice accept *(your carrier)* insurance?

Does this practice have any specialty focuses, such as motor vehicle accidents, sports health, prenatal, pediatric, etc.?

Does this practice offer any supplemental services, such as physical therapy, massage therapy, dry needling, aqua massage, etc.?

Does this practice use manual manipulation and/or other adjustment options (i.e. drop table, activator, decompression, etc.)?
Does this practice offer both treatment plans and single visit options?

Does this practice adjust other joints in the body besides the spine, if needed?

Notes:

Have you already seen a chiropractor but you're not satisfied with the care, return to these fundamental questions and <u>ask them of yourself</u> regarding what you want from your chiropractic experience. Then, adjust these questions to fit your specific situation.

Two of Three Questionnaires

Number:

Address:

Days & Hours of Operation:

Is this practice Corrective or Relief Chiropractic?

Does this practice take x-rays and/or spinal scans?

Does this practice accept *(your carrier)* insurance?

Does this practice have any specialty focuses, such as motor vehicle accidents, sports health, prenatal, pediatric, etc.?

Does this practice offer any supplemental services, such as physical therapy, massage therapy, dry needling, aqua massage, etc.?

Does this practice use manual manipulation and/or other adjust-ment options (i.e. drop table, activator, decompression, etc.)?

Does this practice offer both treatment plans and single visit options?

Does this practice adjust other joints in the body besides the spine, if needed?

Notes:

As you become more and more familiar with the chiropractic way, your needs and desired results may change. As I slowly corrected each area of my spinal misalignments, other areas of discomfort came to the forefront, requiring a shift in my care. Still, these questions provide a great starting point.

Two of Three Questionnaires

Number:

Address:

Days & Hours of Operation:

Is this practice Corrective or Relief Chiropractic?

Does this practice take x-rays and/or spinal scans?

Does this practice accept *(your carrier)* insurance?

Does this practice have any specialty focuses, such as motor vehicle accidents, sports health, prenatal, pediatric, etc.?

Does this practice offer any supplemental services, such as physical therapy, massage therapy, dry needling, aqua massage, etc.?

Does this practice use manual manipulation and/or other adjustment options (i.e. drop table, activator, decompression, etc.)? Does this practice offer both treatment plans and single visit options?

Does this practice adjust other joints in the body besides the spine, if needed?

Notes:

5

Treatment Pitfalls

The Gym Mentality: Practice Makes Perfect

Have you ever seen someone walk into a workout gym looking like they've never been in their lifetime, and then see them walk back out an hour later looking like they've led an entire life of weight lifting? NO! Did that sound like a ridiculous question? Of course, it did because we all know better! It takes time to build up your strength and have the muscles to back it up.

Say someone has a mental illness. Will just one trip to the psychiatrist or therapist resolve everything? NO! This type of treatment takes time to help reshape someone's thought processes.

What about a major illness? Will one session of chemo or dialysis eradicate the disease? NO! It takes several treatments, most of them being a battle in their own right, but we do what we must do to survive.

Now, think about injured backs; the muscles & tendons have to adapt to help continue functioning. Will it take just one visit or one chiropractic adjustment to get it all back to normal? Will those muscles suddenly 'let go' of everything they've known for however long the injury has been at play? NO! Of course not. An injury forces the vertebrae, muscles, tendons, ligaments, and discs into positions unnatural to the spinal structure. Since the body cannot correct this misalignment independently, it instead puts its energy into adapting to the injury. Chiropractic will NOT reverse the injury, and most certainly not after just one adjustment. Chiropractic CAN help, but it can take time.

Chiropractors have the complex and slow task of retraining all of that soft tissue supporting the spine, as intended, versus being stuck in the injury state. The longer the injury state acts as the norm, the longer the treatment will take. It took years to get to where you are right now. One can't possibly imagine all of that can be reversed in a single visit.

Think back to Corrective versus Relief; sure, the relief chiropractor can provide some immediate relief, but it won't take long for the soft tissue to shift back to where it was in the first place. In contrast, a corrective chiropractor will set up treatments with a specific timing between adjustments. As the spine and soft tissue conform to the new movement or location, those visits will become fewer and farther apart. This is the slow and steady corrective approach and is ultimately what saved my life!

By visiting the gym regularly, we aim to get healthier and

stronger. Same with chiropractic! By visiting the chiropractor regularly, we aim to get healthier and stronger. It is not going to take overnight!

The Mall Rat Mentality: The perfect outfit is different for everyone!

Just like in a mall, there are all different types of shops that serve different needs. You might find everything you need in one store, or you may need to go to a couple of places to get the right look that makes you feel your absolute best! Only you know what fit, style, and color will be the right & best options for you!

Also, much like malls, you have the 'big name' stores that have it all in one location, and then there are all the little shops that each do their part. Sadly, the big-name store doesn't actually do it all and has this grand opinion that all the little shops are novelty and cannot ever compete with the other big names. It wouldn't be a mall if it weren't for all those little shops. There would be nothing else to give it that building the hustle & bustle we know.

'Big Medical/Big Pharma, meet Alternative Medicine; I think you two will be a wonderful couple!' It took several years of increased improvement to my spine and overall health before I could convince my medical doctor that chiropractic WORKS! Now, he is educating his other patients on the Wonders of Chiropractic!

Chiropractic is an amazing practice that can unlock so much potential by getting the spine in a state of health. However, it is not for everyone and is not the 'last doctor you'll ever have to go to.' The perfect treatment plan is different for everyone. I implore you to look at the alternatives, get second, third, or eighth opinions, persevere to preserve your health, and be your own advocate.

Cutting Corners

There is no such thing as cutting corners regarding your health! If someone thinks they are "cutting corners' for faster results or quicker improvement, they're not. They are only making the recovery time longer and more difficult.

6

Conclusion

Chiropractic is about helping to heal the spine and, in turn, heal the body. This is why many chiropractors will team up with other professionals to offer a complete and comprehensive experience that can truly unbreak your spirit. After being in pain for 6 years, a short time for some - and I hope this helps you - I finally had hope that I was going to feel better. I wanted off the heavy drugs my M.D.s were prescribing, I wanted to be able to walk without a cane, I wanted to live my life how I wanted to, and I really wanted to show those doctors that I prevailed regardless of their prognosis.

Considering the timing of my accident, you can surmise that I am well past 30 years of age, and guess what?! I am NOT in a wheelchair! The strongest medicine I take for my pain is Ibuprofen and Medical Marijuana. True, I am still in pain, but it is far from what it was when I was still in my injury state.

When I walked into that first chiropractic office, got x-rays taken, and went over my medical history, that chiropractor quite bluntly stated that I should have already been in a wheelchair and he didn't fully understand *how* I was currently walking. I told him it was due to sheer determination and lots of heavy painkilling drugs. Needless to say, I started on a treatment plan. Since then, I have moved and had to find other chiropractors, and throughout the years, I have been to just about every kind there is. From the various corrective types to the relief types. Even after going to a chiropractor for as long as I have, the relief chiropractors almost always set me back in my recovery.

I will tell you that this has been a long journey for me, and it was not always rainbows and unicorns. I had my slips backward. I've sustained new injuries (I still like extreme sports). I've had the wrong adjustments. I've had mindful adjustments. I've worked on specific segments of my spine with various specialty chiropractors. I've even had to resort back to heavier pain medications from time to time. What it all comes down to is that I didn't give up. After so many years of pain, I finally knew how good it felt to feel good, and I don't ever want to go back!

Much like the domino effect of an injury, healing can also be a domino effect. As my spine finally started to heal, other issues that I had been having also started to dwindle. As of today, I can walk, ride my motorcycle, and play disc golf, and I no longer suffer from IBD, kidney stones, recurring/migraine headaches; I don't get sick nearly as often, and the list goes on! I unlocked my body's ability to self-heal!

The most recent development in my health journey, which has been an absolute game changer, is the diagnosis of Ehlers-Danlos, a connectivity tissue disorder. I am so very grateful for having this rare genetic health issue because my accidents could have been much worse if I didn't have the hyper mobility of EDS. This diagnosis has also changed how I get adjusted by my chiropractor. I have not had any major incidents or slips in health since that diagnosis, which was in 2021. So, if you happen to be hyper mobile, be sure to mention that to your chiropractor; it could truly change the entire approach to your treatment!

I hope that my journey helps you along yours!

If you found this book helpful, informative, or entertaining, a positive review on Amazon would be greatly appreciated!

Namaste'

Epilogue

Thank you for reading about my journey and the things I learned along the way.

Keep an eye out for more books about unlocking your true potential through alternative means!

Resources

Professional, C. C. M. (n.d.). Nerves. Cleveland Clinic. https://my.clevelandclinic.org/health/body/22584-nerves

Contributor, N. (2022, May 23). Nervous system 4: the peripheral nervous system – spinal nerves. Nursing Times. https://www.nursingtimes.net/clinical-archive/neurology/nervous-system-4-the-peripheral-nervous-system-spinal-nerves-23-05-2022/

WebMD Editorial Contributor. (2020, November 25). Chiropractor. WebMD. https://www.webmd.com/a-to-z-guides/chiropractor

Chiropractic: in-depth. (n.d.). NCCIH. https://www.nccih.nih.gov/health/chiropractic-in-depth

Rico, S. (2023, July 12). Types of chiropractic adjustments & how they work. Effective Integrative Healthcare LLC. https://www.eihmd.com/2023/02/01/types-of-chiropractic-adjustments-how-they-work/

Organization, C. R. (n.d.). CHIROPRACTIC TECHNIQUES. © 2005 Chiropractic Resource Organization. https://chiro.org/LINKS/ABSTRACTS/Chiropractic_Techniques.shtml

Resource Center - The McKenzie Institute, USA. (n.d.). https://www.mckenzieinstituteusa.org/resource-center.cfm

MSc, N. G. (2023, October 30). Spinal nerves. Kenhub. https://www.kenhub.com/en/library/anatomy/spinal-nerves

Admin. (2019, December 26). CHART OF EFFECTS OF SPINAL MISALIGNMENTS | Ceragemusa. Ceragemusa | Massage Therapy. https://www.ceragemusa.net/modes/attachment/chart-of-effects-of-spinal-misalignments/

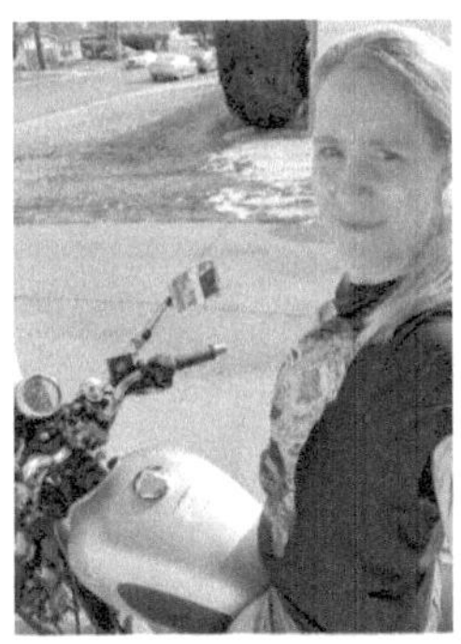

About the Author

Greetings fellow adventures! I am Pearl Fagan. While my love for writing has been a constant companion, I'm thrilled to publish of my first official book!

Over the years, I've written several blogs (under my real name, not my pen name - sorry!) and have created several high level training manuals and programs for government staff within my States taxation units. Please don't hold it against me! For although government training *can* be boring, it's not boring when I am at the helm! Along with writing and document preparation, I've also presented on a gambit of health and wellness topics directly related to spinal health.

I have always had a passion for adventures, of all sorts! I've done things ranging from

   * riding horse as a youth to riding my motorcycle now as a 'real' adult'

* Taking zip-line tours through the Rocky Mountains,

* Participating in Fun/Mud Runs, or

* Taking my Jeep up a mountain pass that nobody else would dare to go!

* And by biggest adventure yet: being a mom!

Finally, I have the deep desire to help people! When I found chiropractic and learned that my life wasn't over at 23, I wanted to sing it from the top of the Mount Lindo. Chiropractic not only changed my life but ignited a burning desire to share its wonders with the world. I even started working for chiropractors as a marketing specialist, public outreach manager, and event coordinator!

What can I say, I get passionate about the things that impact me and I want to share it with the world!